TEST

This book is designe
optimisation therap
dictionary, and so you ....
between some of the chapters. You may w....
read it from start to finish, or you may prefer to
dip in and out to read the areas that most concern
you. You may end up doing both. The choice is
yours.

Ross Tomkins has written a practical and
immensely useful book on hormone optimization
for aging men. It is comprehensive and easy to
follow. Ross provides an excellent overview of the
symptoms of low T so that men can recognize this
slow process and take action, and gives a wide
ranging overview of all of the biohacks men use to
boost testosterone.
Dr. Judson Brandeis
Board Certified Urologist & Sexual Medicine Expert

After researching TRT for around a year I was
delighted to come across Alphagenix and the
opportunity to have a Doctor supervised treatment.
The service and communication has been excellent
from my day one initial enquiry through to my
treatment. I would highly recommend Alphagenix to
anyone seeking help, advice and treatment for TRT.
Alphagenix Patient

Now 11 months with Alphagenix on a safe dose of
TRT and it's been amazing. My mood, energy levels,
limbo, weight loss and muscle gain have all improved.
I honestly feel like I'm in my early 20's again but with
a few more wrinkles. The support from Alphagenix is
one of the most important things to me. Knowing if I
had any question no matter how stupid it may seem
to you, someone will answer you on the same day
(usually within a couple of hours). I look forward to
being with Alphagenix for a very long time and can't
thank them enough for making me whole again.
Alphagenix Patient

AGEING
AND THE
ANDROPAUSE

Reclaim Your Youth with Testosterone Replacement Therapy

Ross Tomkins

purple star publishing

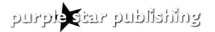

First published in Great Britain 2023 by Purple Star
Publishing

Design by Clare McCabe www.purplestardesign.co.uk

ISBN13: 9798851450198

DISCLAIMER

Dedication and Thanks

This book is dedicated to all of the men out there who feel like I felt 11 years ago.

I would not have written this book without the unwavering support of my amazing wife Joanne. She is the rock at the centre of our family and has helped me to explore and refine my own approach to health and wellbeing; from Wim Hof breathwork in the Lake District and having conversations with a Shaman in Central America, to everything else in between, including hormone optimisation.

In fact, throughout our 19 years together, she has backed most of my crazy ideas and we've shared the successes and failures of those decisions as a family unit, along with our two beautiful children, Izzy and Lincoln. They too, continue to inspire and push me to be the best example of a human being in every area of life I can be, every single day. Thank you.

Thank you also to Steven Kuhn and Lane Belone whose Humble Alpha coaching programme helped me to find my voice in the Men's Health space, and to realise that my own feelings of insecurity had prevented me from sharing my hormonal journey until today.

I offer sincere thanks to Dr Bernard Willis for diagnosing my testosterone deficiency all those years ago, and for setting me on this path. And finally, a huge thank you to my epic business partner, Ben Paglia, who has made the last four years in business the most fun yet.

Onwards and upwards Pagsy!

CONTENTS

Part 3 – Living an optimal life 77

Part 1

Testosterone and TRT

1.

My story and why "Ageing And The Andropause" exists

Do you feel a little different than how you did a few years ago? You probably aren't sure exactly why.

This story begins 11 years ago when I realised that I didn't feel myself anymore. If you are reading this book, there's a good chance you can identify with this. You probably can't explain how you feel different, let alone why. There's just this underlying, gnawing and unsettling feeling that something has changed.

If you've not noticed it yourself yet, others around you may have. Perhaps your partner, your best mate, your colleagues or your doctor have made jokes about you becoming grumpier, less fit, less tolerant and put it down to you getting older.

I can certainly relate. After relaying my symptoms to him, my first NHS endocrinologist told me that everything I was experiencing was 'in my head'. There's nothing to make someone feel more paranoid and more alone than telling them that their symptoms aren't real.

As a qualified physiotherapist, I wasn't prepared to settle for this answer. Over the years I've sought for answers to that "off" feeling with an inquisitive, clinical mind. I've explored countless different healing modalities, diets, exercises and treatments.

These include, but are by no means limited to yoga, Pilates, meditation, mindfulness, HIIT training, weight training, running, cycling, bioresonance, hypnosis, sensory deprivation, hyperbaric champers, Wim Hof breathwork and cold immersion, clarity breathwork, sacred plant medicines, acupuncture, massage, Reiki, Seichem, halotherapy, crystal therapy, red light therapy, paleo, ketosis, the Autoimmune Protocol and more supplements and shakes than I can count.

I've also seen doctors, coaches, personal trainers and shamans on 6 continents, and perhaps, some of what I have learnt from them will make it another book one day. However, possibly the most valuable teachings I have taken away from my exploration, and the purpose of this book, is the need for Hormone Optimisation Therapy.

Hormones are most often associated with women, but the reality is that men have hormones too. And just like for women, they play an important role in our health and wellbeing – so much so that my symptoms didn't start improving until I had a much better understanding of the fine balance of our body system that is responsible for hormone production and distribution – the endocrine system.

This book is going to focus on one hormone in particular. It's one that most people have heard of but is rarely discussed in a positive light. In fact, you could even say that talking about it is something that some men consider taboo. This hormone is testosterone.

Testosterone is a hormone found in both men and women and is vital for maintaining optimal health in both sexes. However, this is particularly the case for men, who can be severely affected by sub-optimal levels of testosterone. Low energy, reduced muscle mass, poor mental focus, depression, low self-esteem, insomnia, weight gain and even erectile dysfunction have all been linked to low testosterone levels.

Over the next few chapters, we're going to explore testosterone in greater depth, including looking at what can happen when testosterone levels fall. We'll also look at methods you can use to boost your testosterone levels, counteract the symptoms you may be experiencing and improve your overall health. We call this Hormone Optimisation Therapy, and it is a relatively new area of medicine which means you may not find many doctors practising it or referring patients to it in the NHS.

Important note about terminology

During this book, you'll see me referring to a number of important terms. I'd like to briefly introduce and clarify these now.

Hormone Optimisation Therapy or HOT is a super-new term that many people aren't familiar with. Nevertheless, it's something that I believe will become a much more recognised term in the not-too-distant future. It will refer to a tailored treatment plan that is designed to restore depleted testosterone levels, balance other hormone levels and take other positive steps to counteract the symptoms of low testosterone so that men can live life optimally. Essentially it is a holistic approach to male wellness.

Testosterone Replacement Therapy or TRT is a specific treatment that can be taken as a standalone solution to low testosterone, or form part of HOT. It refers to different therapy types, all of which will boost your natural testosterone levels. Examples of forms of TRT include patches, gels and injections.

Hormone Replacement Therapy or HRT is a similar term that you've almost certainly heard of in relation to menopausal women, but essentially, HRT also applies to men. The only difference is that the main hormone being replaced is testosterone rather than oestrogen.

2.

What is testosterone and why is it important?

Testosterone is a hormone that is found in both humans and animals. However, it is the major sex hormone in males and plays a variety of important roles in both the growth and development of boys, and later in adulthood. This is because it's the main androgen – a hormone that gives men their 'male' characteristics. Testosterone is responsible for things like:

- The development of the penis and testes
- The deepening of your voice during puberty
- The development of facial and body hair during puberty
- The loss of hair that can be experienced in later life
- Bone growth and strength
- Muscle size and strength
- Sex drive
- Sperm production
- Mood and behaviour

Testosterone is present from birth, but the levels change throughout your lifetime. Male testosterone levels rise drastically during puberty, which account for many of the changes listed above. However, testosterone tends to peak around the age of 18 or 19, before declining throughout the rest of adulthood [1].

According to guidelines from the British Society of Sexual Medicines, the 'normal' range for testosterone in the UK is 8-30 nmol (nanomoles per litre)[2]. This is clearly a wide range, with low testosterone considered to be less than 8 nmol. **However**, an OPTIMAL testosterone level is 20 nmol and above.

3.
Being better than normal

One of the problems with medicine is that all too often, medical practitioners and happy to settle for "normal". Normal blood pressure, normal cholesterol, normal blood sugar, normal testosterone. While the term "normal" may be applicable, do you really want to settle for normal? Because in most cases, normal means that something is ok, average, even mediocre. Unfortunately, "ok" is forgettable. If you watch a movie that's mediocre, you probably won't watch it again, or recommend it to your friends. If you eat a meal that's mediocre, you might not return to that restaurant, and you almost certainly won't order that dish again.

Don't you want to strive to feel better than just normal? What if you could feel strong, empowered, even elite? What if you could be the best husband, father, friend, businessman and person you could be? With HOT, the goal is to achieve optimal health and wellbeing, not just "normal".

4.
Generational testosterone decline

Now before you start to panic about dropping hormone levels, it's important to understand that the decline of testosterone is nearly always slow and steady. You aren't going to wake up one morning with a balding head, paunch and no sex drive.

However, the gentle decline in testosterone levels can mean that it is more difficult to spot, and this can make any developing symptoms all the more frustrating. You might not automatically link a little weight gain or thinning hair to testosterone, but inside your body, that hormone is responsible for much more than you expect.

Many doctors and health professionals believe, as I do, that there's nothing normal or healthy about the side effects that come with depleting testosterone levels. In fact, there is mounting evidence to suggest that there is also a generational decline in the amount of testosterone than men today have – as much as 1% per year[3].

Exactly why this is happening is thought to be a combination of factors, from increasing obesity and more sedentary lifestyles to higher stress levels and exposure to more external toxins that can interfere with the body's hormones, such as those found in plastic bottles and other packaging, skincare products and some detergents[3]. And with products containing many ingredients, often with long and complex names, we routinely don't realise we are exposing ourselves to these toxins until after the damage has been done.

While your dad and your grandad probably had testosterone levels that were higher at aged 20 than yours were, it doesn't mean that you have to live with the effects of low testosterone.

5.
What is Andropause?

In this book, you'll hear us talking about the term 'andropause'.

This is a very real term that's been recognised by the National Institute of Health and comes from the word "Andras" in Greek, which means human male, and "pause" which is a word used to describe cessation. It is, to all intents and purposes, the male equivalent of the female menopause in that is it defined as a syndrome associated with a decline in feelings of wellbeing caused by low levels of testosterone in older men.

6.
Does the male menopause really exist?

So, let's get one thing straight from the off. The male menopause, also known as the andropause, testosterone deficiency, secondary hypogonadism and probably many more names that I've not included here, is a very real thing. However, it's also still very poorly understood, often misdiagnosed and absolutely still a taboo subject.

This probably doesn't come as much of a surprise. After all, it takes a great deal of time, effort and research for scientific community to allow a new concept to exist. Often a continuous cycle of testing, argument, debate, trials, analysis, more debate... the reality is that even some of our most widely accepted, modern medical theories took years to progress from conjecture to accepted fact.

When it comes to andropause, there's no getting around the fact that we are still in the early stages of scientific acceptance.

Not everyone is on board with it... yet. But new evidence is coming to light all the time. Nevertheless, this is a bit of a moot point for men and their partners who have already identified their condition and taken positive steps to treat it.

I'm one of them. I have experienced the amazing effect that testosterone restoration has had on me after I went through a long period of feeling very low and unlike myself. And I want you to be able to recognise it in yourself and seek help quickly, so that you don't have to live with the effects of andropause for any longer than necessary.

Fact: Men just don't talk enough about their worries

It's an unfortunate fact that many more men suffer from low testosterone than are diagnosed with the condition. One of the main reasons for this seems to be our reluctance to talk about our worries and our feelings. For a long time, men have been perceived to be les 'in touch' when it comes to their feelings, and I can't necessarily say it's an argument that I disagree with.

Despite some degree of progress over the

last few decades, men speak much less about mental health than women do.

A large part of this stems from traditional masculine role socialisation which has made many men feel that their masculine identity conflicts with showing emotion. Research from men's health charity Movember, found that nearly a third of men feel pressure to be masculine[4].

To maintain this perception of manliness, the research also found that 38% of men don't talk to others about their feelings, and a whopping 3 in 10 haven't ever cried or shown extreme emotion in front of others.

Unsurprisingly, all of that repression isn't good for us. When we are already battling with low mood and poor self-esteem, bottling up our emotions only drives both of these things even lower. And the frustration of being in a constantly low state drive us to 'act' rather than talk – often leading to rash, impulsive and even selfish behaviours in a bid to try and pull ourselves out of the pit of depression that is trying in vain to suck us back in.

Perhaps then it shouldn't be of any surprise that our nearest and dearest don't recognise the symptoms of low testosterone as anything more than the grumpiness, mood swings and withdrawal that accompanies older age. After all. Most people associate the symptoms we'll be displaying – low energy, apathy, tearfulness and a loss of interest – with clinical depression [5].

As we know, anything related to men's mental health is generally considered taboo and far too many men still won't seek help, even if their low mood and feelings of hopelessness are severe enough for them to consider self-harming or even suicide. You've probably heard this statistic before, but it doesn't hurt to share it again so I will.

Suicide is the biggest cause of death in men under the age of 50.

Let that sink in. Not talking, not sharing our worries is literally killing us. If we don't get help when times get tough, we are more likely to have suicidal thoughts and we are more likely to be successful in taking our own lives. In contrast to a few generations ago, we've generally become a little better at demanding answers to the personal problems that we face, but there's a lot of work to be done before we can say we're out of the deep water. We still have a great deal to learn about refusing to suffer in silence, and society has a long way to go to fully accept and embrace that men have mental health struggles too, for us to be able to trust those we choose to confide in, and for it to truly be ok for men **not** to be ok.

At the end of this book, I'll signpost to some charities and organisations that may be of use if you are struggling with your mental health, and you need a discreet and non-judgemental ear or shoulder.

Why is the male menopause seldom diagnosed in men?

It's not just women who suffer from fatigue, low libido, mood swings, loss of focus and concentration and a whole raft of other issues in midlife. The truth is that men can experience each and every one of these things, including night sweats, during their middle years. For women, it's the lack of oestrogen that accompanies menopause that causes these symptoms. For men, it's caused by a drop in the normal production of testosterone. One of the most important differences is that menopause causes a fairly sudden and drastic change in their hormone production, while for men, the decrease in testosterone production is significantly more gradual.

So, why is the andropause so rarely diagnosed in men? One of the main reasons for lack of diagnosis is the difficulty with which andropause can be identified. The gradual decrease in testosterone means that the effects can be tricky to pinpoint at first and seem to relate entirely to psychological and lifestyle factors, rather than physical ones.

We're also more likely to try and distract ourselves from what is happening inside our body by focusing on the things that we can control – namely our behaviour. Sadly, our choice of distraction is often destructive. We may throw ourselves into work at the expense of our family, friends or health. We may become gamblers, make reckless decisions and even become sexually promiscuous. We're also more prone to substance abuse than women are [6].

Another reason why andropause may be much less diagnosed than menopause is because health professionals simply don't know what to do about it. Hormone Optimisation Therapy – or HOT for short – is a fairly new area of medicine. Like me, many men who have finally sought help and visited doctors to discuss their symptoms have found them dismissive.

Those doctors that are aware of it have generally been slow to accept it, and even slower to refer patients to the Hormone Optimisation Therapy that I have found to be a complete game-changer.

Isn't it just a midlife crisis?

You've probably heard countless jokes about having a midlife crisis as you've got older. The term was actually coined by a Canadian Psychoanalyst called Elliott Jacques back in 1965, who used it to describe some of the common behavioural changes that men typically go through in mid-life. Buying a sports car, having an affair and dressing like someone 20 years younger may be mid-life clichés, but they are also very demonstrative of the impulsive and potentially destructive behaviours we've listed above.

However, the jokes about a midlife crisis are a lot less funny when it's you that is faced with the stereotypes of middle age - when you notice you are starting to lose muscle definition and you're six pints away from a beer belly, when your hairline starts to recede or man-boobs don't only affect Steve at the pub but in fact are staring back at you in the mirror and making you rethink your wardrobe choices.

And don't even get me started on the loss of libido or, those occasions when you are up for some quality time with your partner, but your old boy isn't having any of it. Sheesh. You probably won't be surprised to learn that it's estimated that only 33% of men who have erectile dysfunction issues seek help and advice [7].

All of the things we've listed above, and a whole lot more, happen in midlife. That's because this is also when the andropause kicks in.

Andropause is different for everyone

Once you accept that andropause is a very real condition, and it's likely you are in its clutches, it's also important to be aware that how andropause affects you might be very different to someone else. Dr. Bernie Willis, a medical practitioner who is fully conversant in the hormonal changes that come with age and has years of experience in Hormone Optimisation Therapy in both men and women says "I've learned over the years that everybody's different – there is no one-size-fits-all.

Just as when women go through the menopause, 80% may show some symptoms, whereas the remaining 20% will sail through without having any problems at all".

So, what affects how severely you experience andropause and the symptoms you get? Genetics seem to play a large role, as well as the balance of your other hormones, not just testosterone. Again, it comes back to this balance of hormones we've talked about before. Dr. Willis compares hormones to instruments in an orchestra. "They all need to work in tandem. If one member of the orchestra is out of tune, the other instruments can't play properly".

While many men may mistakenly believe that Testosterone Replacement Therapy is the only solution for andropause, Dr. Willis believe that jumping straight to TRT is a mistake. Instead, he advocates Hormone Optimisation Therapy as the best place to start. This is because HOT focuses on restoring and rebalancing all of your hormones, rather than simply adding extra testosterone into the mix.

The curse of the midlife moobs

At this point, it's worth briefly mentioning one of the most common side effects of low testosterone – gynecomastia. Better known as "man-boobs" or "moobs", it refers to excess fat that develops in the chest area. The reason for the development of midlife moobs is quite simple.

When testosterone production decreases, muscle mass begins to deplete too and when this happens, what was previously muscle can turn to fat. When you combine this with increased levels of oestrogen, it's pretty normal to see some breast tissue growth.

Moobs are even more likely if you are already overweight or obese. This is because oestrogen is stored in fat cells. The more fat cells you have, the more oestrogen you have in your body, and so the more likely you are to experience the side effects of high levels of oestrogen.

The easiest way to tackle moobs is to combine HOT with a healthy, protein-rich diet and plenty of exercise. Once your weight is under control and your hormones are perfectly balanced, the any existing excess breast tissue should start to disappear.

7.

The dangers of environmental toxins and hormone disrupting chemicals (xenoestrogens)

Before we go any further, it's prudent for us to spend a couple more minutes looking at oestrogen in further detail too. Oestrogen is often overlooked when it comes to male health. Nevertheless, it plays a critical role in your overall health and wellbeing.

Oestrogen is one of the main female sex hormones, although it does occur in men in small amounts. Like testosterone, oestrogen is responsible for the development of typically female characteristics, such enlarged breasts and increased fat stores. However, a particular form of oestrogen called estradiol is important for male sexuality, specifically for modulating your sex drive and maintaining erectile dysfunction[8].

Some of the other functions of oestrogen in men include:

- Improving bone health and aiding bone development during puberty, while also protecting your skeleton in later life by reducing the risk of osteoporosis (brittle bones).
- Boosting cardiovascular health by increasing healthy cholesterol (HDL), lowering unhealth cholesterol (LDL) and reducing total plasma cholesterol.
- Increasing neurological health and reducing the chance of stroke by protecting neurons and stimulating the creation of new ones.

Xenoestrogens are a synthetic compound that mimics the effects of natural oestrogen, can boost its production and disrupt the delicate balance of hormones within the body.

They can be found in all sorts of products from food and skincare to insecticides and building supplies. The following list is by no means exhaustive but contains just some of the hormone disrupting chemicals to look out for.

Hormone disrupting chemicals in skincare

- 4-Methylbenylidene camphor (4-MBC) commonly found in sunscreens.
- Parabens (methylparaben, ethylparaben, propylparaben and butylparaben) commonly used as a preservative.
- Benzophenone commonly found in sunscreens.

Hormone disrupting chemicals in industrial products and plastics

- Bisphenol A or BPA (monomer for polycarbonate plastic and epoxy resin) an antioxidant in plasticisers.
- Phthalates, in plasticisers.
- DEHP, plasticiser for PVC.
- Polybrominated biphenyl ethers (PBDEs) flame retardants used in plastics, foams, building materials, electronics, furnishings and motor vehicles.
- Polychlorinated biphenyls (PCBs),

Hormone disrupting chemicals in food

- Erythrosine / FD&C Red No. 3
- Phenosulfothiazine, a red dye.
- Butylated hydroxyanisole / BHA, a food preservative.

Hormone disrupting chemicals in building supplies

- Pentachlorophenol, a general biocide and wood preservative.
- Polychlorinated biphenyla / PCBs, found in electrical oils, lubricants, adhesives and paints.

Hormone disrupting chemicals in insecticides

- Atrazine, found in weed killer.
- DDT, a banned substance found in some insecticides.
- Dichlorodiphenyldiphenyldichloroethylene, a breakdown product of DDT (above).
- Dieldrin
- Endosulfan
- Heptachlor
- Lindane / hexachlorocyclohexane, also used to treat lice and scabies.
- Methoxyclor
- Fenthion
- Nonylphenol and derivatives (industrial surfactants, emulsifiers for emulsion polymerisation, laboratory detergents and pesticides).

Other Hormone disrupting chemicals

- Propyl gallate, an antioxidant added to some foods.
- Chlorine and chlorine by-products.

- Ethinylestradiol, found in the combined oral contraceptive pill.
- Metalloestrogens, a class of inorganic xenoestrogens.
- Alkylphenol, found in cleaning detergents.

So, why so you need to be aware of the dangers of hormone disrupting chemicals and xenoestrogen? Well, just like all other hormones, the balance of oestrogen alongside your other naturally-occurring hormones needs to be just right for optimal health and wellbeing. Too many hormone disrupting chemicals in your body could disrupt this balance and may lead to many of the side effects associated with andropause. Some studies have also implicated xenoestrogens as potential contributors to the development and progression of prostate cancer [9].

How to reduce your exposure to xenoestrogens

While oestrogen is naturally occurring, there are things that you can do to limit your exposure to xenoestrogens and which may make it easier to keep your oestrogen at an optimal level and prevent it from having a negative impact on your day-to-day life.

Check your personal hygiene products

As we know, xenoestrogens can be found in many personal hygiene products. You can help reduce your exposure by being vigilant when it comes to choosing your products. Check labels for the toxic chemicals we've listed above and be particularly on the lookout for parabens and phthalates, which are very commonly used in the cosmetic industry.

Thanks to an increasing awareness of the toxicity in many personal hygiene products, there are more chemical-free varieties available than ever before. Look for chemical-free soaps, shampoos and toothpastes. If you want to use scented products, look for those which are made with natural-based fragrances such as essential oils.

Reduce your exposure to pollutants

Pollutants are all around us. You may not even be aware that you are being exposed to them on a daily basis. You can take steps to reduce your pollutant exposure by:

- If you smoke, cutting down or quitting altogether.
- If you live with someone who smokes, ask them to smoke outside to limit your exposure to second-hand smoke.
- Check the labels of your household cleaning products, detergents and more for signs of toxic chemicals listed above and swapping them for a chemical-free alternative.
- Using glass and/or ceramic containers to store food instead of plastic ones.
- Avoid using your microwave as much as possible.
- Don't microwave plastics, as this can cause some of the BPA to leak out.
- Avoid placing plastic bottles in direct sunlight as this too can cause BPA to leak out.
- Don't refill plastic water bottles.

Reduce the number of xenoestrogens in your diet

The best way to reduce the number of xenoestrogens that may be entering your body through your diet is to choose organic, pesticide-free fruit and vegetables wherever you can, and to wash them thoroughly before consuming them. If you do need to eat nonorganic produce, peel the skin before you cook/eat them. Where possible, you should also opt for hormone-free meat and dairy products.

While reducing the number of xenoestrogens you are exposed to is no guarantee that you won't experience the effects associated with increased oestrogen levels, it could make it more likely that you will avoid them.

What are the symptoms of low testosterone and how is it measured?

Testosterone levels are measured through blood tests, which makes actually determining how much testosterone you have in your body a fairly easy process. As we know, most doctors believe that anything less than 8 nmol per litre 2 is considered low testosterone. However, studies estimate that as many as 40% of men over the age of 45 will have levels that come in below that range [10].

Blood tests to measure testosterone should usually be performed in the morning between 7 and 10am. That's because during these hours are when your testosterone is typically the highest. Just as a little addition, this may also explain why many men are generally more up for sexual activity in the mornings rather than the evenings!

Symptoms of low testosterone

No two men with andropause are the same, and so while we are going to look at some of the most common symptoms of the condition, it's important to be aware that you may not experience all of them, and the severity of the symptoms that you do experience can also vary.

The symptoms of low testosterone can be categorised into physical, psychological, cardiometabolic and sexual.

Physical symptoms
- Low energy and fatigue
- Decreased muscle mass and strength
- Reduced physical performance and slower recovery post-exercise
- Joint aches and pains
- Sleep disturbances
- Hot flushes and sweats
- Decreased body hair and hair on your head
- Gynaecomastia (man-boobs)

- Reduced bone density meaning breaks are more likely

Psychological symptoms

- Irritability
- Unexplained sadness
- General low mood
- Low motivation
- Loss of interest in things that you were involved in before
- Poor concentration
- Impaired memory
- Brain fog
- Low self-esteem

Cardiometabolic symptoms

- Weight gain / obesity (a BMI of 30 or higher)
- Increased abdominal fat
- Metabolic syndrome
- Insulin resistance, prediabetes or type 2 diabetes

Sexual symptoms

- Erectile dysfunction
- Reduced libido
- Infertility
- Small testes

- Delayed ejaculation
- Decreased frequency or absent morning and night time erections

If you are reading these symptoms and nodding along with any of them, I recommend that you fill in the Androgen Deficiency in Ageing Males (ADAM) questionnaire which you can find either in the appendix of this book, or on our website https://www.alphagenix.co.uk.

The ADAM questionnaire is a straightforward and internationally recognised and accredited assessment tool that is often used by doctors to help diagnose testosterone deficiency, and which may help you when it comes to discussing your symptoms with your doctor.

Your doctor may go on to use the Ageing Males Scale (AMS) and/or the International Index of Erectile Dysfunction IIIEF) to evaluate the severity of your symptoms and monitor the improvements over time. You can find the AMS and IIEF-15 are available in the appendix of this book.

8.
Testosterone Replacement Therapy (TRT)

Testosterone Replacement Therapy, or TRT as its commonly referred to, it a common treatment recommended for men with testosterone deficiency. TRT can be prescribed as a standalone treatment, or in the case of Hormone Optimisation Therapy, it's usually undertaken alongside other positive, hormone-balancing lifestyle steps to maximise the likelihood that you can achieve optimal results.

What are the benefits of TRT?

There are many different benefits associated with TRT. These can typically be divided into physical, psychological, cardiometabolic and sexual function benefits.

Physical benefits of TRT

TRT has been consistently proven to improve body composition in males by increasing lean body mass and decreasing body fat [11]. This in turn helps to improve muscle strength, athletic performance and recovery. Other physical benefits associated with TRT include improved bone density, reduced blood pressure, better overall cardiovascular health and even higher quality sleep [12].

Psychological benefits of TRT

There's plenty of evidence out there that demonstrates the improvement in mood that is associated with TRT too. Many men report that after starting TRT they experience less anxiety, more energy and improved mood with fewer mood swings [12].

Cardiometabolic benefits of TRT

Diabetes is a common risk factor in men during middle-age, particularly during andropause. However, evidence suggests that TRT has a beneficial effect on insulin sensitivity, glucose control and lipid profile, all of which can reduce your risk factors for developing Type 2 diabetes [12].

Sexual function benefits of TRT

Low libido and sexual dysfunction are among the easiest and most reversible symptoms of low testosterone. Many men report that TRT helps them to rediscover their sex drive and improves the quality of their erections, both of which can contribute to greater overall satisfaction when it comes to your sex life. These effects are further heightened when TRT is combined with the use of phosphodiesterase 5 inhibitors like Viagra.

Is TRT safe?

As with most therapies and medical treatments, there are some risks associated with TRT. I firmly believe in being empowered to make informed decisions about our health and wellbeing, and for this reason, it's important that I share a little about these risks with you. However, it's also essential that you are aware that your level of risk should be assessed by your doctor *before* you start treatment, and not everyone is automatically a suitable candidate for Testosterone Replacement therapy.

While studies indicate that only a relatively small number of men experience side effects from TRT [13] the reality is that side effects are extremely rare provided that your testosterone levels are in the optimal range. There have been reports of men taking too much testosterone replacement – such as to try and build excessive muscle mass - and it is this action that can lead to significant side effects [14].

It's important to be aware that TRT can also lead to a reduction in sperm production. Therefore, your fertility could be affected by going onto Testosterone Replacement Therapy. If you are considering having children in the future, you should discuss this with your doctor prior to starting treatment [15].

How long does it take for TRT to start working?

The good news is that if you do start TRT as part of Hormone Optimisation Therapy, you can expect to see results fairly quickly. Although the exact speed of the effects of TRT can vary between individuals, most men start to see an improvement in their symptoms and a positive effect on their quality of life within three or four weeks of starting treatment [16].

Improvements in sexual function and libido typically take a little longer, with most men needing to take TRT for up to six months before they see the maximum benefit in this area of their life [16]. Similarly, research suggests that it can take around six months for men to achieve their optimal wellness goals, including reaping the full physical, emotional and sexual benefits of TRT treatment.

Does TRT have anti-ageing properties?

We'd all like to turn back the clock on the ageing process. Recent studies have found that testosterone increases the production of an enzyme called telomerase [17]. Telomerase is an enzyme found in cells that helps keep them alive. It does this by preventing regions of repetitive DNA sequences at the end of a chromosome, called telomeres, from shortening. It's a bit like how the plastic ends on shoelaces prevents them from fraying early on and increases their longevity.

Research has found that telomere length, which can be affected by various lifestyle factors, can also affect the pace of ageing and the onset of age-associated diseases. Shorter telomeres have been associated with increased incidence of diseases and poor survival. By preventing telomeres from shortening, it's thought that TRT has a mild, anti-ageing effect.

Part 2

A deeper look at the symptoms of low testosterone and how to take back control

While we've covered the key symptoms associated with low testosterone briefly above, it's now time to gain a much deeper understanding of them – how and why they happen, the effects that fluctuating testosterone levels have on your day-to-day life and, most importantly, what techniques and tools you can use to take back some control.

The most important thing to be aware of is that in some way, shape or form, all of these symptoms and the steps you need to take to get your life back on track are interlinked. For this reason, you will see a degree of cross-repetition in the recommendations that we make.

9.
The physical effects of low testosterone

We already know that the physical effects of low testosterone are some of the most noticeable, while also being some of the most concerning for men experiencing them.

Improving falling energy levels

One of the most obvious areas of your life that may be affecting by diminished testosterone is your energy levels. Now, you almost certainly experience periods of fatigue anyway. Unless you are lucky enough to have a lifestyle that leaves you far removed from many of the stresses and strains of the world, you'll already be used to peaks and troughs of energy that align with your day-to-day activities.

You'll be well used illness being followed by days or even weeks of sluggishness as your body takes the time it needs to recover. This is especially true as you get older, as it takes longer for us to 'bounce back' from the things that affect our body and mind.

So, when is low energy more than simply a by-product of a busy life? If you feel that you are in a good place physically and mentally, are eating a healthy, balanced diet, getting regular exercise and sleep for at least seven hours every night but you are **still** waking up feeling groggy, unmotivated and just not quite ready to participate in life, it could be a good idea to get your testosterone levels checked.

The thing is, as you get older, many changes happen inside your body. You can't see them, but they are happening nonetheless, and it's the effects that you'll experience that will let you know that they are. Higher levels of fatigue are just one consequence of andropause.

Feeling too tired for any between-the-sheets action all of a sudden? As we've discovered, testosterone plays a key role in libido, and many men experiencing low levels may find that their sex drive starts to reduce – something which can be frustrating for both partners in your relationship.

So, what can you do to help counteract the effects that reducing testosterone has on your energy levels? Here are a few suggestions to help you get back in control of your vitality.

Pace yourself

Take a step back and look at your week. How busy and stressful is it really? Are there things that you can do to reduce the mental and physical burden of your day-to-day life and help you to get more accomplished in a shorter time frame? If looking at your diary fills you with dread, it's time to cut down on your commitments so that you don't psychologically shut down before the week begins. And pacing yourself in the day will help you avoid burn out, reduce your stress levels and make sleep come more easily.

Work on improving your sleep pattern

Testosterone is principally made while you are asleep. However, sleep is also the time when the rest of your body relaxes, resets and makes ready for the next day. There's a reason that a doctor tells you to sleep as much as possible following a surgery. If you aren't getting enough sleep, you are compromising your body's ability to recover from any trauma, and to make enough testosterone to keep your natural T levels well-balanced.

The good news is that there are tried and tested techniques proven to help you both fall, and stay, asleep. These include:

- Limiting stimulants like caffeine, nicotine and alcohol before bedtime.
- Don't do any exercise before bed either, as the endorphins will keep your body alert rather than wearing you out ready for sleep.
- Try not to use your phone or any other digital device for at least an hour before you go to sleep as blue light emitted by digital screens is shown to block a hormone called melatonin that makes you tired. Bright light can also wake you up and make it hard for you to fall back asleep.
- Make your room cooler. Your body temperature naturally changes as you fall asleep, so going into a cooler environment can make it easier to feel tired.

Take a look at your diet

Food is the fuel our body needs to function. However, the quality of the fuel you are putting in can directly affect your energy levels. Think of it a bit like choosing whether to put unleaded or super unleaded petrol into a performance vehicle. Standard fuel will get the car where it needs to go but using super unleaded will give the engine what it needs to deliver optimal performance. If you owned a Ferrari, you'd want to put the fuel in it that keeps it running optimally. Why should your body be any different?

We all know what a healthy diet means – plenty of fruit and veg, low saturates fat, lots of protein and minimal sugar and alcohol. However, sticking to a consistently healthy diet is hard, and for many of us, it's not until we really start to feel the impact of poor eating habits, or we experience a health scare that we start to realise just how important it is to eat well. If you are experiencing fatigue, fuelling your body right can give your energy levels a much-needed boost.

Book an appointment with your GP

If you've implemented the steps above and you are still struggling with tiredness, or if you are generally just concerned about the severity of your fatigue, it's important to schedule an appointment with your GP. There are many health conditions that can directly affect your energy levels, including thyroid issues, sleep apnoea, diabetes and even the side effects of some medications. Your GP will vary out any necessary tests to rule out other underlying causes for your low energy levels.

Preventing muscle loss and maintaining your physique

Do you look at younger guys and wonder how they manage to stay so lean, despite eating what they like and spending little time at the gym? The answer could lie in their testosterone levels. Testosterone helps build muscle mass, making it much easier to maintain a fairly lean physique.

However, when your androgen receptors (responsible for binding male hormones to muscle cells) don't get enough of this hormone, your muscle cells can't maintain your muscle fibres and they begin to degrade. In the absence of testosterone, the hormone oestrogen steps in and replaces areas of muscle with fat. In short, a six pack can quickly become more of a flapjack if it's not addressed quickly.

Unfortunately, muscle loss often swiftly follows dropping energy levels in the pecking order of andropause symptoms. When the two are combined, it makes it particularly difficult for men to implement the changes needed to get their physical appearance back on track. This is especially true when you factor in the psychological impact of diminished muscle loss.

So, what can you do prevent muscle loss?

Get regular exercise

Unless you've been living under a rock, you'll know that exercise is one of the best ways to build muscle mass, or in this case, reverse lost muscle due to a drop in your testosterone levels. Combining cardio like running, swimming or cycling with resistance training should deliver the best results, keeping your heart healthy and keeping your muscles toned and strong.

However, while exercise can help you to build muscle, it doesn't actually counteract your dropping testosterone levels, which will continue to fall unless you consider a treatment like hormone optimisation therapy. It'll be a bit like pushing jelly uphill. All first doing exercise to minimise muscle loss may feel easy, but over time, it will get harder and harder to keep muscle loss at bay. The ideal solution is to boost your testosterone levels by making sure you get plenty of sleep, eating well and opting for hormone optimisation treatment and combining that with regular exercise to counteract muscle loss and keep yourself in physically great shape.

Successfully maintain a healthy weight

As we know, when a man experiences low testosterone levels, it is difficult for him to build or maintain muscle. Muscle weighs more than fat, which is why some extremely muscly men – like Dwayne 'The Rock' Johnson – are medically considered to be overweight even though they have very little body fat. However, muscle also requires a great deal of energy for you to maintain it. The more muscle mass you have, the faster your body will burn calories to fuel it. When muscle starts to break down, your metabolism will slow. This means that if you are still eating the same number of calories as before, any excess 'fuel' will be turned into stubborn pockets of fat.

Men tend to store excess fat in the upper part of their body, including their abdomen and chest. We've already mentioned the prevalence of man-boobs in andropausal men in the previous chapter. Meanwhile, excess fat on the abdomen creates the 'beer belly' effect that so many men struggle with, and that puts you at risk of additional health problems due to the accumulation of visceral fat around your organs.

When muscle turns into fat you might find that not only do you look less lean, but that the scales start to shift in an unfavourable direction. You may have already been carrying some excess weight or find that weight gain seems to happen much faster, despite no real changes to your eating habits.

Now, obviously if you are already overweight, it's a good idea to address this to optimise your overall health and wellbeing. However, simply cutting back on calories probably won't cut it, so instead it's a good idea to speak to your doctor before starting any sort of weight loss regime. They'll be able to advise you how to create a balanced nutrition plan that will support your goals without leaving you starving hungry, battling cravings and likely to give up altogether within a few weeks. You should also explain to your doctor that you believe that your weight gain is a result of low testosterone levels. They can assess this and confirm a diagnosis, which will help you to decide what you need to do next to take back control of your body – much of which includes the advice already offered in this book such as testosterone replacement therapy, more sleep and positive nutrition.

If you are already a healthy weight, suddenly cutting back calories isn't going to make much difference to your physical appearance. Instead, it's important to follow a healthy, balanced diet and activate the other methods of boosting your testosterone so that you can keep your body in the best physical shape possible.

Overcoming sexual dysfunction

Probably the biggest taboo for many men is the effect that low testosterone can have on their libido and sexual performance. Although low testosterone alone rarely causes erectile dysfunction, the other effects of a drop in this hormone can contribute towards your ability to get in the mood for sex, or to experience an active and fulfilling sex life.

The important thing to remember is that for men, the ability to get an erection is as much mental as it is physical. It doesn't matter how much you try to manually arouse yourself, if your head isn't in the game, it's going to prove difficult to develop an erection that is hard enough to enjoy penetrative sex, or to experience climax yourself. Low mood, low self-esteem and lack of energy can all affect your sex drive before you take into account any physical effects you may be experiencing.

As we get older, we are also at greater risk of developing cardiovascular problems. Many people are surprised to learn that there is a very strong link between erectile dysfunction and heart disease. Since the arteries in the penis are so narrow, erectile problems can be one of the first warning signs of heart disease and a future heart attack.

If you are experiencing erectile dysfunction, it is always advisable to speak to your doctor as they can rule out any serious underlying causes, such as cardiovascular disease. They can also perform a blood test to check your testosterone levels to determine if they are low and this could be contributing towards your low sex drive or erectile difficulties.

Many men are relieved to know that they are not alone in experiencing a loss of libido or sexual dysfunction after their testosterone levels start to wane. They are even more relieved to discover that, in addition to testosterone replacement therapy which obviously works to restore testosterone levels, there are other treatments that can help.

Focused shockwave therapy

Shockwave therapy may sound unpleasant and even dangerous, but it is a safe and clinically-proven treatment for erectile dysfunction, with a success rate of more than 75% [19].

Shockwave therapy involves passing high frequency waves through the skin to treat a wide range of different disorders, including erectile dysfunction. Treatment is fast, painless and discreet with virtually no risks or side effects, and you can get back to your usual daily activities right away after each session.

In erectile dysfunction, the high frequency

waves stimulate blood flow to the penis, making it easier to get and sustain an erection. They also stimulate tissue repair and regeneration; helping to grow new blood vessels in the penis which will also support future erection capability.

Viagra (and other PDE5 inhibitors)

You'll certainly have heard of Viagra. You may have also heard of other similar medications called Cialis, Levitra and Tadalifil. All of these are what are known as PDE5 inhibitors and work by improving the blood flow to certain tissues, including the tissues of the penis. By increasing blood flow to the area, it makes it easier to get and sustain an erection. Studies have found that PDE5 inhibitors like Viagra can keep working for up to five hours after being taken, making it possible to enjoy prolonged sexual activity.

10.
The social and emotional effects of low testosterone

Many men are surprised to learn just how much of an effect depleted testosterone levels can have on their mood and behaviour.

Addressing your mental health

Despite countless campaigns and awareness days, there is still so much stigma around mental health and wellbeing, especially when it comes to men. As we discussed in the previous chapter, suicide is the biggest cause of death in men under the age of 50, and around three quarters of deaths from suicides each year are men. Yet, for many reasons, many of us are still reluctant to let people around us know when we aren't coping well with day-to-day life.

How do I know if I have depression linked to testosterone deficiency?

Depression causes a variety of different symptoms, some of which are obvious and others which are harder to attribute to low moods. Some of these symptoms include, but aren't limited to:

- Feelings of emptiness, numbness and hollowness
- An inability to find joy in things that you once took/found pleasure in
- Feeling anxious, stressed and physically unwell at the thought of the future
- Difficulty maintaining concentration for even a short period of time
- Memory loss, brain fog and other cognitive disruption
- Sleeping all the time, and feeling perpetually tired
- Weight that yo-yos up and down
- Feeling worthless or guilty
- Feeling as though you want to harm yourself/actually self-harming
- Suicidal thoughts

Depression is a serious illness and if you

experience any of the symptoms above, it is essential that you find someone you can talk to be it a friend, family member or a healthcare professional. Regardless of whether your depression is caused by low testosterone or something else, getting help is crucial.

There are many different types of depression and many of the symptoms of low testosterone mirror those of clinical depression. However, as with all mental health conditions, it's important to speak to a medical professional to try and determine the underlying cause of your feelings.

For men experiencing low testosterone, their low moods are often a reflection of the effects of their condition on their day-to-day lives, such as coping with unhappiness about the changes to their physical body, or the impact of dropping testosterone levels of their sex life. Similarly, anxiety and other similar feelings may affect them in the same way.

While antidepressant and anxiety medications can certainly help you to regain some degree of equilibrium, many men are reluctant to take them or worry about the side effects or long-term impact of their use. If your mental health concerns are caused by low testosterone, engaging in hormone optimisation therapy can be a very helpful alternative since it will work to address the underlying cause of your anxiety and depression rather than simply mask it. This is because, as we know, testosterone replacement therapy effectively takes over your testosterone production, inhibiting the production of natural testosterone in your testicles, and replacing it with a synthetic alternative. As a result, it's not an option that you can dip in and out of. Instead, TRT requires ongoing commitment, not least because the process can impact your natural fertility and so should only be considered if you've got no plans to have any more children.

Managing stress

Do you wake up with a knot in your stomach in the morning? Feel sick when you look at your bank statement? Can't sleep through worry about a family member or friend who is sick? Whether it's related to work, family, money, health or something else entirely, stress is another major contributor to low mood, anxiety and depression, as well as being something that can have an actual physical effect on your health.

Managing stress isn't easy, particularly when

various sources of stress accumulate at once – that old saying of things happening in three's has to come from somewhere after all! Talking therapies can be particularly effective when it comes to managing stress that is contributing towards anxiety and depression. When stress levels are under control, it becomes much easier to handle the other problems that life throws at us. So, by taking steps to manage your stress, you may find managing the symptoms of your low testosterone becomes easier.

Coping with low self esteem

It's probably unsurprising to hear that many men who are in testosterone decline suffer from poor self-esteem. This low self-esteem can result from a combination of the physical changes and mental changes caused by the change in their hormones, including:

- Muscle loss and build-up of fat in areas that were previously lean
- Having to work harder at the gym than before
- Loss of libido or sexual dysfunction
- Difficulty coping with stress
- Brain fog and poor memory
- Mood swings

The impact of having low testosterone won't only affect you, but it will also have a wider effect on your friends and family. After all, if you feel like crap about yourself, you aren't exactly going to be the life and soul of the party. In fact, you probably won't even want to go to the party in the first place. And it can be desperately upsetting for your loved ones to see you lose your confidence and your personality fade.

Boosting your self-esteem won't be an overnight process, but there are things that you can do to help you gradually rediscover your inner light. These include getting plenty of sleep, cutting out alcohol and making time to exercise every day – something that will increase your natural endorphins. Getting outside into nature has been proven to help boost mood, since increased oxygen helps your brain and body to function more optimally.

And of course, getting out into the sunshine provides us with much needed vitamin D – something which many of us are lacking and which is essential for strong, healthy bones and muscles and has shown to be important for a healthy cardiovascular system.

You should also consider meditation and

yoga, both of which are reliable tools in stress management, but which can also help you to improve your mood and see things from a new perspective – both of which can be invaluable for improving the way you view yourself.

Banish brain fog and boost cognitive function

Ever found yourself completely zoning out from the task in hand? One minute you'll be hyper-focused on an activity and the next, you'll have forgotten something basic like how to spell a word or what someone's name is. You might feel like a fool, but brain fog is a very normal side effect of low testosterone levels.

Your brain is the most complex part of your body, and it relies on a perfect balance of chemicals, hormones and other substances to function optimally. Just like physical abilities diminish with advancing age, so too do your cognitive ones.

However, if you find that confusion, memory loss and other cognitive functions start to fluctuate in your 30s and 40s, it could be that your testosterone levels are to blame. Visiting a GP will help rule out any other underlying causes and allow you to get on with the business of boosting your testosterone levels and getting your brain cells back on track.

Unsurprisingly, all of the therapies for testosterone-enhancing listed in this chapter can help you to banish brain fog, from eating right and drinking plenty of water, to getting at least seven hours of sleep every night. Many men also find that hormone optimisation therapy perfectly combines with these techniques to maximise their effect and the positive impact they have on their quality of life.

Part 3

Living an optimal life

When it comes to this world, unless you believe in reincarnation, you'll accept that we only get one life. Living it to the max should therefore be at the very top of your priority list. What you consider an optimal life, and what someone else does may differ, but one thing that everyone has in common is that it's almost certainly necessary to be healthy and happy to achieve it.

11.
Longevity medicine and heart health

Longevity medicine is advanced personalised preventive medicine where the outcomes are determined by our longstanding lifestyle choices. The better the choices we make, the more likely we are to be able to live a full and optimal life.

Meanwhile, making negative choices such as smoking or drinking excessive alcohol consumption are more likely to lead to disease and poor outcomes.

Much like the andropause itself, there's no one-size-fits-all approach to longevity medicine. It's also a fast-emerging field which means that many doctors may not have even come across it yet, let alone be actively able to offer you the support you need to implement longevity medicine in your life.

There are predominantly three factors involved in longevity. These are:

1. Genetics
2. Lifestyle
3. Environment

Genetics

Unfortunately, genetics is one aspect of longevity medicine that we can't control. Research suggests that siblings and children of long-lived individuals (people who have lived to a fairly long age) are also more likely to remain healthy for longer and to live to an older age than their peers. For example, people aged 70 with centenarian parents are less likely to have the age-related diseases that are common among other people their age [20].

Fortunately, genetics is just one element of longevity, and it may not necessarily be the defining factor. Scientists are now speculating that for the first 7 or 8 decades of life, lifestyle is a much stronger determinant of health and longevity [20].

Lifestyle

Lifestyle choices are one of the most predominant causes of health problems. They are also one of the common threads in whether or not someone is likely to reach a significant age. Scientists have been studying people aged 90 and over as part of a longevity study, in order to determine what factors have contributed to their long lives. Key similarities between them included being non-smokers, a healthy weight and coping well with stress. Their healthy habits made them less likely to develop conditions like high blood pressure, heart disease, diabetes and cancer than their peers.

The good news is that how we have a choice in our lifestyle. We can choose to smoke or not smoke. We can choose to have a glass of whisky or a few pints every night, to drink alcohol only when it's a special occasion, or to not drink it at all. For most of us, we have the ability to control our weight, make sure we get plenty of exercise and enough sleep at night.

Now, that's not to say that any of these things are easy. Not everyone is blessed with a fast metabolism that means that they don't need to watch what they eat. Some people are under excessive amounts of stress through no fault of their own – such as the breakdown of a marriage, a sick partner, or problems at work.

The most important thing is to have realistic expectations and not to be too hard on yourself if there are days or weeks when you can't make healthy lifestyle choices. We're all human and nobody can be expected to make the best choices all of the time. **But**, if we try and make sure that the majority of our lifestyle choices are good ones, we too reduce the risk of illness and disease, and increase the likelihood that we will experience a long, healthy and active life.

Environment

Our environment has also been shown to play a role in longevity. Environmental improvements in the early 1900s, such a better availability of food and clean water, improved housing and living conditions and better access to medical care, dramatically extended the average lifespan [20].

There are many ways in which the environment contributes towards, or harms, our health and wellbeing. For example, the World Health

Organization has reported on the link between specific diseases such as stroke, ischaemic heart disease and chronic obstructive pulmonary disease (COPD) and air pollution [21]. Meanwhile, background radiation – which is predominantly from things like X-rays and CT scans but can also occur due to high levels of Radon in the ground, has been shown to contribute to higher levels of lung cancer. In fact, much of Cornwall, England, is designated as a radon-affected area and Cornwall Council have a section of their website designated to this [22].

There are limited steps we can take to control the environment around us, but where we can, we should carefully consider whether we could potentially be putting ourselves in harm's way.

12.
Heart health

Cardiovascular/heart disease are the terms used to describe any medical condition that affects the heart or blood vessels. On average, men develop heart disease 10 years earlier than women do [23].

Unfortunately, research is starting to show a link between low testosterone levels and heart disease, as well as type 2 diabetes. In fact, erectile dysfunction is well-cited as an indicator of potential cardiovascular problems later on. The reason for this is that the arteries of the penis are much smaller than those in the heart, and as a result, any arterial damage often occurs in the penis long before the heart is affected. Men in their 40s who have erection problems but no other risk factors for cardiovascular disease run an 80% risk of developing heart problems within 10 years [23].

Of course, other factors such as obesity, excessive stress and high cholesterol can also contribute towards an increased risk of problems with your heart health. There's good news in that heart disease is preventable by living an optimal lifestyle and managing your risk factors.

Here are 6 of the most effective ways of strengthening your heart health.

1. Get regular exercise. Your heart is a muscle too, and exercise will make it stronger.
2. Give up smoking. Smoking is one of the biggest contributing factors in cardiovascular disease.
3. Maintain a healthy weight. This may mean losing weight through a combination of diet and exercise first.
4. Eat a heart-healthy diet. Healthy fats are proven to be good for your heart. Some foods containing healthy fats that you should consider adding to your diet include avocados, dark chocolate, oily fish like salmon and mackerel, nuts and chia seeds.
5. Don't overeat. Eating a lot of food at once causes blood to shift from the heart to the digestive system, and trigger faster and irregular heart rhythms, which could lead to heart failure or a heart attack.
6. Don't stress. Stress is far from just a psychological problem. Instead, it causes a very real, physical reaction including

raising blood pressure, sometimes to very dangerous levels. Chronic stress has also been linked to other health conditions, including obesity, diabetes and Alzheimer's disease.

13.
Testosterone Replacement Therapy and PTSD

At this point, I would also like to talk briefly about the newly emerging link between TRT and Post-Traumatic Stress Disorder, better known as PTSD.

The link is a bit of a conundrum. Firstly, research shows that 80% of men who have PTSD (or, incidentally, have suffered a traumatic brain injury), suffer from low testosterone [24]. However, the inverse is also true in that men with low testosterone have also been found to be more at risk of developing PTSD.

Most people have heard of PTSD. What many people don't realise is that PTSD can develop after a single serious traumatic event, such as a car accident or serious injury/illness, or following prolonged exposure to trauma, such as sexual abuse in childhood. Since individual responses to trauma can vary significantly, there's no clear way to predict who may develop PTSD and who won't.

In one study from the U.S, a 29 year old male Marine veteran who has been suffering with PTSD for many years despite taking medication and undergoing cognitive behavioural therapy, was tested for various hormones including thyroid, adrenal, gonadal, IGF-1 and prolactin. He was discovered to be experiencing testosterone deficiency and started on TRT. Within weeks of beginning treatment, the veteran reported improved sleep, better energy levels, increased sexual function, better concentration, strength and endurance. Most importantly for him, his irritability and explosiveness were replaced with an increasing sense of calm and tolerance for others. He even began to go to get his groceries during peak hours – something which he has previously avoided doing in favour of night time visits so as not to trigger any outbursts. These notable improvements continued for more than a year thanks to testosterone supplementation.

14.
Measuring biomarkers in Hormone Optimisation Therapy

Biomarkers are biological molecules found in blood, other body fluids or tissues. Essentially, they are characteristics of the body that can be measured to give your doctor a good idea of your overall health. Biomarkers play a crucial role in early diagnosis, disease prevention, deciding which drugs to prescribe and monitoring how well different medications work.

Measuring your biomarkers is an important part of any Hormone Optimisation Therapy treatment plan. These biomarkers will be measured alongside analysing your hormones, insulin sensitivity, longevity testing (mentioned above) and a physical examination will help guide your doctor in creating your bespoke HOT plan.

There are many different biomarkers – some which are more important for men's health than others. In the appendix of this book, you'll find our basic biomarker test which contains information about the 43 biomarkers that are most important for men to live optimally.

15.
Further optimisation: Biohacking

When you hear the term 'hacking' you probably think of computers, emails and cybersecurity. 'Biohacking' is a slightly different concept and refers to changing your body's physiology and biochemistry through science and experimentation with different tools, techniques and supplements with the aim to increase your energy levels and vitality. Without getting too crazy and discussing things like implant technology and genetic upgrades, it mainly focuses on lifestyle and dietary changes, along with the use of wearable technologies like FitBits and Apple watches, which provide reminders telling us when to move, when to eat and when we need to get more sleep.

Personally, I love biohacking and, as I mentioned at the start of this book, over the years I've tried all sorts of tools and methods to optimise my health. In fact, I'm still constantly looking at the newest and most innovative ways of increasing my health and happiness. I'm particularly interested in anything that can increase energy, improve tissue healing and promote longer life, and I'm not put off by a lack of scientific evidence. If something is safe and low risk, it's game on for me.

In the following few paragraphs, I'll talk about some of the biohacking methods that I've tried and are working well for me, in the hope that you too could find them useful.

Blue light blocking glasses

One biohacking tool that is becoming increasingly popular is blue light blocking glasses. Blue light is all around us all of the time. In fact, the sun is our primary source of blue light, and we need some blue light for optimum health. It helps balance our circadian rhythm (our sleep-wake cycle), boosts alertness, elevates mood and improved memory and brain function.

However, too much blue light has been linked to a range of unpleasant symptoms such as blurred vision, eyestrain, difficulty sleeping (if you are exposed to too much blue light before going to bed) and headaches. Research has even found that it may contribute towards conditions such as diabetes, obesity, heart disease and even come cancers [26].

Blue light can spell problems for your long-term vision and eye health too. Long term exposure could damage the cells of the retina (part of the eye that is responsible for sending messages to your brain to tell you what you can see), and contribute to cataracts, age-related macular degeneration, growths on the eye (called pterygium) and eye cancer [27].

I recently had a long discussion with both an optician and a general practitioner about the usefulness of blue light glasses at protecting the eyes against the blue light that is emitted by our digital devices, like our phone screens and laptops. Neither healthcare professional had any positive supporting evidence to say that the glasses would be effective at helping to improve my sleep. However, neither did they have any evidence that they could be harmful.

In fact, they both agreed that the worst possible case scenario for blue light blocking glasses is that they don't work. My personal view is that, in the absence of long-term data for this relatively new concept, and with the general consensus that they aren't harmful, what have I got to lose by wearing them? As a result, blue light blocking glasses have made it into my daily routine and I now wear them every day for a couple of hours before bed.

Cold immersion therapy

Like many people, I first came across cold immersion therapy when I heard about The Iceman, Wim Hof. However, the truth is that the health benefits of cold water immersion and cold therapy are not a new concept. Almost 2500 years ago, the ancient Greek physician Hippocrates claimed that it cured lethargy, while more recently, in the 19th century, American Founding Father Thomas Jefferson claimed his good health was a result of bathing his feet in cold water every morning.

Wim Hof has certainly boosted awareness of cold immersion in the 21st century, combining it with breathing exercises and meditation to create the 'Wim Hof method' – which has countless followers around the world.

Much like blue light blocking glasses and other bio hacking techniques, scientific evidence for its success is sketchy. Nevertheless, there is an abundance of experiential and anecdotal evidence. When you combine this with the fact that cold immersion therapy is a technique that has endured millennia, where other 'health fads' (such as the vibrating belt in the 1960s, and the Thighmaster craze of the 1990s) have been and gone, it certainly adds weight to its effectiveness. And with athletes regularly citing the benefits of cold water exposure as an effective recovery strategy and new studies being undertaken all the time, it seems like it's only a case of when and not if the benefits of this biohack will be scientifically confirmed.

Heat/sauna therapy

Like cold water immersion, saunas and exposure to intense heat for therapeutic effect has also been around for a long time. More recently, infrared saunas have gained popularity among biohackers worldwide. Both traditional and infrared saunas have been linked to a wide range of health benefits including detoxification, faster metabolism, weight loss, increased blood circulation, pain reduction, skin rejuvenation, boosted immune function, better sleep and stress management, and more [28].

Saunas work by triggering a process called vasodilation. Vasodilation is essentially increased blood flow around the body, and this helps to dissolve toxins floating around in your bloodstream so that they can be processed out of your body naturally (through the usual methods of excretion – urine, faeces and sweat). Under the heat provided by a sauna, your body also releases endorphins which can lessen pain and improve your mood.

Red light therapy

You've probably heard of Seasonal Affective Disorder, or SAD as it is more commonly known. SAD is a type of depression that has a seasonal pattern, usually occurring during the winter months when the days are shorter, the nights draw in earlier and the weather is colder. The two main symptoms associated with SAD are low mood and a lack of interest in life.

One of the main, and most commonly accepted treatments, for SAD is red light therapy. Sometimes referred to as RLT, red light therapy is exactly what it says on the tin – the use of red light to create a therapeutic effect. While it's not a substitute for natural sunlight, it has a range of health benefits that mimic those provided by the sun including boosting your mood and energy, accelerating healing and increasing circulation. There are also a range of skin benefits associated with red light exposure, such as reduction in fine lines and wrinkles, reduced stretch marks, improved skin texture and help with conditions like rosacea and psoriasis [29].

Red light therapy is thought to work by producing a biochemical effect in the cells of your body that improves your metabolic and nervous system processes and supports overall health and wellbeing.

You can buy red light therapy equipment for home use, but I would recommend that you seek the services of a private clinic offering this therapy.

Viagra – not just for erections

Viagra may be the most commonly prescribed medication for erectile dysfunction (along with Tadalafill, another popular ED drug, but I firmly believe that in the not too distant future, they will also be routinely prescribed as part of a Hormone Optimisation Therapy treatment plan for men over 40 years old. Not only is Viagra an extremely safe and effective drug for sexual dysfunction, but studies also suggest that men who take these medications are less likely to experience heart failure, stroke and a heart attack [30]. With these medical issues being an increasing risk for men after the age of 40, a small, daily dose of Viagra could be all that is needed to significantly increase the likelihood that we can continue to live full and healthy lives. The fact that the drug can also help us to maintain erections, which in turn keeps our penis healthy and enables us to continue to have a fulfilling sex life is an added bonus!

Intermittent fasting

This section of the book wouldn't be complete if I didn't mention intermittent fasting. A hot topic and a widely debating bio hack, intermittent fasting is a very popular and successful eating plan that is effective for both weight loss and weight management [31].

So, what is intermittent fasting and how do you do it?

Intermittent fasting, as the name suggests, it an eating plan that sees you follow a schedule of both eating and fasting at very specific times. If you have followed any sort of in the past, you'll know that calories and food groups are core principles in most of them. However, with intermittent fasting it's less about what you eat and more about when you eat. With intermittent fasting, you'll only be eating at specified times, and will be fasting for a certain number of hours every day, or perhaps just eating one meal on a couple of days each week. The underlying premise of intermittent fasting is to stimulate the body to burn fat.

Mark Mattson, Profession or Neuroscience at John Hopkins University, completed pioneering research into the way that the brain responds to fasting and exercise. His 25 year study uncovered the specific ways in which intermittent fasting slows the ageing process, reduces the risk of diseases such as obesity, diabetes and Alzheimer's, and improves both brain and body performance [32].

It's not news that obesity is on the rise and people today find it much harder to maintain a healthy weight than our ancestors did. Thousands of years ago, back when dinosaurs roamed the earth and people had to hunt for food, they were adept at being able to survive for long periods between meals as it could sometimes be days before they could catch or gather the food they needed to survive.

Even as recently as 50 years ago, people ate less frequently. With less convenience food available, there was less snacking, and as TV finished at 11pm, people went to bed rather than staying up binging the latest Netflix series or playing games online. The reality of the 21st century is that we could stay awake, and therefore eat, 24 hours a day if we wanted to.

Approaches to intermittent fasting

There are a number of different approaches to intermittent fasting, but all of them have one thing in common – you choose a set schedule of times of when you are allowed to eat, and when you need to fast. One popular approach is to limit eating to a period of eight hours every day, and then fast for the remaining time. Some people prefer to just one meal a day on two days of the week. It's about finding an intermittent fasting plan that works for you.

From his study, Mattson found that when the body goes without food for many hours, it uses sugar stores first, before then burning fat to fuel itself. He refers to this process as metabolic switching. This pattern, Mattson comments, is in contrast to the normal eating pattern of most American and indeed UK people, which largely consists of grazing throughout the day. Intermittent fasting will prolong the time between meals, so that your body burns through the sugars in the food you've most recently eaten and begins to burn fat to continue to function.

In his research, Mattson discovered that it could take between two and four weeks for the body to get used to intermittent fasting. However, like with all diets, you could find yourself feeling tired, hungry and cranky until your body adjusts. The key is to stick it out and get through the difficult period to reap the benefits. For many people, finding this willpower is the hardest part.

Examples of intermittent fasting plans

- One of the most popular intermittent fasting approaches is the 5:2 plan. This involves eating normally for five days each week, and then limiting yourself to a single meal of no more than 600 calories on the other two.
- Some people prefer the daily approach. This is where you restrict yourself to only eating food within a six or eight hour

window each day, and then fasting for the remaining hours. Many people say that this is one of the easiest intermittent fasting plans to follow.

• Some people like to try and fast for longer periods, such as 24, 36 or even longer hours. However, there's no evidence to suggest that this is any better for you, and it's likely to be much harder to maintain. Some experts suggest that if you don't eat for a really long time, your body might start to store and preserve fat as a response to the threat of starvation.

What to eat when you are intermittent fasting

One of the first questions anyone has when they are starting a diet/healthy eating plan is "what can I eat" and intermittent fasting is no exception.

When you are fasting, surprise surprise, you aren't allowed to eat anything at all. You can drink black coffee, black tea or any beverage that has zero calories.

When you aren't fasting, it can be tempting to go crazy and eat whatever you want. You didn't eat for 16 hours or whatever after all, right? Wrong. If you spend the eight hours you have to eat stuffing in crisps, biscuits and junk food, you aren't going to get the nutrition you need for optimal health, and there's still a good chance you'll put on weight, not to mention cause a spike in your blood pressure. Experts like Mattson recommend that you eat a normal range of food that includes unrefined/complex carbohydrates, healthy fats, leafy greens and lean proteins.

Benefits of intermittent fasting

There is plenty of research being done around intermittent fasting. Some of the listed benefits include, but aren't limited to:

- Improved thinking and memory
- Better blood pressure
- Lower resting heart rates and other heart-related measurements
- Better maintenance of muscle mass
- Increased endurance
- Weight loss
- Reduced risk of type 2 diabetes, or improvement in people with the condition

Is intermittent fasting safe?

It's important that you check with your doctor before starting any new diet or eating plan. However, generally intermittent fasting is not recommended for:

- Children and young people under the age of 18
- Pregnant or breastfeeding women
- Anyone with Type 1 diabetes who is taking insulin to control their condition
- People who have or have previously suffered from an eating disorder

If you have any concerns about your suitability for intermittent fasting, always speak to your doctor.

16.
Meditation

While I could have included meditation under biohacking, but the immense power of this technique means that I think it deserves a space in this book all of its own.

As we've already discovered, stress plays a huge role in our hormonal health. During times of stress, the adrenal glands produce an abundance of cortisol – a stress hormone that regulates a wide range of processes throughout the body, including metabolism and immune response. High levels of cortisol cause a 'fight or flight' response in us and lowers our testosterone production. I know the cliché is that men think about sex all the time, but the reality is that when we're under immense amounts of stress, it's often the last thing on our mind.

Now, don't get me wrong. Some cortisol is essential. It converts proteins into energy and reduces inflammation. However, chronically high levels of cortisol are **not** good for our bodies. Over time, it can cause hormonal imbalances, impair cognitive function, trigger digestive issues and even weaken our immune system [33]. Put simply, chronic stress is bad for our health.

While we can't always control what is happening around us, we are always in control of our own actions. One of the best things we can do to help manage stress is to meditate.

Many men in particular are keen to disregard meditation as a bit 'hippy' or a bit 'woo'. However, when it comes to getting stress under control, it's scientifically proven to be successful [34].

You won't be surprised to hear that meditation isn't anything new. People have been doing it for thousands of years, sometimes as part of their religious or spiritual beliefs, but also often simply as a way of calming their mind and improving their overall wellbeing.

The concept of meditation is simple. It's training your attention to achieve a mental state of calm concentration and positive emotions. Exactly how you do this can vary, as there are many different techniques that can be used to achieve this heightened state of awareness and attention. With practice, you can learn to relax your mind and allow stressful thoughts to fade away.

Getting started with meditation – 3 simple steps

One of the easiest ways of getting started with meditation is to listen to your breathing.

1. Start by sitting comfortably, closing your eyes and focusing on your breathing.
2. Breathe in through your nose and out through your mouth, but don't focus on changing the length or depth of your breaths.
3. Try and ignore any thoughts that pop into your head and concentrate fully on your breathing, feeling air coming into your body and expanding your lungs, and then leaving your body.

By practising daily, you can gradually work your way up to longer and longer sessions. Optimally, you should aim to meditate for between 15 and 30 minutes every day, or whatever your schedule allows.

Apps for meditation

It's the 21st century, there's an app for everything, and meditation is no exception. These apps will help guide you through different techniques and styles of meditation, although with so many to choose from, it may take a while to find the best one for you. Some of the most popular include Calm, Insight Timer, Headspace and The Mindfulness App.

The Consciousness Ladder

Many people are surprised to learn that there are different levels of consciousness. The aim of meditation is to climb the consciousness ladder to reach some of the highest levels.

When your conscious mind is fully functioning and awake it is referred to as being in a 'beta' state. In a high beta state, the brain is extremely aroused and overactive. A prime example of this is someone who is a fight or flight mode due to excessively high levels of endorphins.

The first stage of meditation aims to reach the 'alpha' state of consciousness. This is where you are relaxed, calm and lucid, but not thinking. The voices in your head begin to quiet.

The deeper you can relax into this state, the more likely you are to be able to reach the 'theta' level of consciousness. This is deep relaxation that enables enhanced retrospection, mind and body healing and more.

Finally, the 'delta' level is the deepest state of unconsciousness and dreamless sleep that goes beyond meditation. This is where you want to be when it comes to falling asleep at night. However, many men find it difficult to fall asleep and when this happens, it's usually because their mind is working overtime.

Exactly what is keeping you awake at night could vary, from problems at work or planning for the next day, to things happening with friends, family or your health. Overthinking is the arch nemesis of a good night's sleep. Unfortunately, it can also create an imbalance in the neurotransmitters like serotonin and dopamine in your brain, harming your memory and your emotions. Many people become trapped in a cycle of overthinking and negative thoughts that prevents them from climbing the consciousness ladder and getting adequate rest.

Meditation, especially when practiced before bed, is a great way of quieting an overthinking brain and preparing for good quality sleep. Some people also like to meditate in the morning, to clear their mind of any negative thoughts and energy so that they feel refreshed and ready to start the day with a clean slate.

Imitating the sleep-wake cycle

I briefly touched on the sleep-wake cycle, also known as your circadian rhythm, in the part of this book where we looked at blue light blocking glasses. Going to sleep at night isn't something that we are taught to do. It's an impulse – something that we've been doing every day since we were born. Changes in the environment and our own body rhythm sets the pace for our sleep-wake cycle. As we lie in bed at night, melatonin (a night-time neurotransmitter) will move our brain waves from a beta state to an alpha state, then to a theta state and finally a delta state, putting us into deep sleep. When the sun starts to rise, serotonin (a daytime neurotransmitter) reverses the process and beings us through the states of consciousness back to being awake again.

When we decide to meditate, the action of closing our eyes trigger the start of a change in the chemistry of our brain to stop serotonin and start melatonin instead. Essentially, we are tricking our body into preparing for the next state of consciousness. As we sit calmly, with our eyes closed, we can slow and then stop intrusive thoughts, block out sensory details and reach the calmer, more relaxed state that can help to reduce our stress levels, manage our emotions and improve our overall health and wellbeing.

Types of meditation to consider

Meditation comes in many different forms and what works for one person may not work for another. For this reason, I recommend that you don't simply try one and give up, but instead persevere to find the form that works most effectively for you. Personally, I find it very hard to quiet my mind and I can't even cross my legs, let alone get into a half-lotus position, so I prefer mindful walking in nature, which never fails to provide respite from my daily life.

Here are some other forms of meditation that you may like to consider:

- Zen meditation
- Mantra meditation

- Transcendental meditation
- Yoga meditation
- Vipassana meditation
- Chakra meditation
- Qigong meditation
- Sound bath meditation
- Focused attention meditation
- Body scan meditation
- Visualisation meditation
- Mindful walking meditation
- Nature bathing meditation
- Reflective meditation
- Loving kindness meditation

Once you find the one that works for you, practice regularly and just let the magic happen.

17.
Habits and habit stacking

Why have I included habit stacking in a book about TRT? Because, like many of the other elements I have included in this chapter, you need more than simply TRT to make positive and optimal lifestyle choices. And since the vast majority of our lifestyle choices come down to habit, there's pretty much no way I could write this chapter without including a section on ditching bad habits that could be comprising our health and building good ones.

You might not think that you have any habits at all, but I can guarantee you do, you just don't realise it. Our habits make up a large part of who we are and how we live our lives. And they aren't always big, obvious choices either. Many people think that a habit is going for a run every Saturday morning, always ordering the same food from the Chinese takeaway or biting their nails. But the reality is that if we make the same choices time and time again, that's a habit. Reading a few pages of a book before going to sleep every night is a habit. Scrolling on your phone when you go for a morning poo is a habit... you get the picture!

The thing about habits is that no matter what type they are, good or bad, healthy or unhealthy, they can actually have a big impact on our happiness. They can shape our actions and attitudes and our ability to make decisions.

Stating the obvious here, it's a good idea to always build positive habits. But to do that, we first need to understand how habits are formed and how to recognise any mistakes which could lead to us developing bad ones. By examining a little of the science that lies behind making habits, we can have better control over those that we develop.

So, what is a habit?

A habit is something that you do because you have developed an inclination to do it. It could be helpful, harmful or indifferent. Good habits help us to achieve our goals and make us feel proud of ourselves. Bad habits can have the opposite effect and be destructive and even shameful.

Habits largely come down to a chemical in our brain called dopamine. Dopamine is considered to be a 'reward chemical', as its release is driven by reward-seeking behaviour. Dopamine plays a crucial role in mediating the reward value of things like food, drink, sex, social interaction and substance abuse[35]. Dopamine often has a specific trigger or number of triggers for each individual. For example, you may smell cigarette smoke and immediately want to reach for a cigarette yourself. If stress causes you to pour a glass of wine to help you unwind at the end of the day, you will quickly automatically turn to a glass of wine after any stressful event.

Here are a few examples of the types of habits that many of us have:

- Automatically fastening our seatbelt when we get into a car
- Reaching for a cigarette or sugary treat when we are stressed
- Biting our nails when we are anxious
- Tapping our foot when we are feeling impatient
- Playing with a pen or doodling when we are bored and restless

From your brain's point of view, setting up habits is making your life more efficient.

Effectively, you are able to do these things subconsciously, so without actually thinking about them. For some habits this is great news for your health and wellbeing – such as if you automatically remember to bend using your knees and not your back, or if you always go for a run before work. Other habits, like twiddling your hair, biting your nails or stress eating are more damaging.

Habit stacking is a special form of habit-forming and involves identifying a current habit you already do each day, and then stacking your new behaviour on top. In doing this, it can make the new and improved habit easier to remember.

Aren't habit and routine the same thing?

Many people confuse a habit with their daily routine, and it's easy to see why. After all, both involve doing certain things over and over. However, the key difference between the two is awareness. A routine is something that needs deliberate thought and input to maintain it, like remembering to stack the dishwasher or making a packed lunch every morning. A habit is a subconscious action that you may not even be aware of until someone else points it out to you. To make a routine a habit, it needs to move from being planned to intuitive.

The science behind habit-forming

Habit forming is a fairly simple process that happens in a cycle that is often referred to as a habit loop. Coined by the author of "The Power of Habit", Charles Duhigg, a habit loop is considered to be at the core of every habit we develop, no matter what it is. There are four stages to every habit loop, and these occur in exactly the same order every time.

1.   The Trigger
We continually analyse our environment to find any clues as to where a reward-seeking activity may be found. For example, a packet of biscuits left on the side, or a colleague nipping outside for a smoke. This clue will trigger your brain to begin the habit loop and move to the next stage.

2.   The Craving
A craving is the motivational force that occurs behind each formed habit. It is your craving that will drive you to act and take the step needed towards the next stage in the habit loop.

3.   The Response

This refers to the performance of the habit –
eating the biscuit, having a cigarette etc. It
also refers to the thought and decision not
to give in to the reward-seeking action if you
are trying to fight against a bad habit, like
smoking.

4.   The Reward

The reward is the ultimate goal of all and any
habitual behaviour and the final stage in the
habit loop. And once the rush of dopamine
subsides, your body will automatically move
back to stage 1 and start looking for a new
trigger again. For people wanting to give up a
habit, the lack of reward is what makes giving
it up so difficult as the desire isn't fully sated.

How long does it take to establish a habit?

There have been many studies carried out on
habit-forming, and there's no set answer as to
how long it will take to establish a habit. For
people who have addictive personalities, a
new habit can form extremely quickly – within
as little as 18 days. However, for others it can
take as much as a year. The general consensus
is that 59 to 70 days is the average time it
takes to form a new habit [36].

The main factor that can affect habit formation times is motivation, such as the motivation to diet for a special occasion, or to give up smoking before a big birthday.

Avoid these five mistakes

Here are five mistakes that you should try to avoid when you want to replace a bad habit with a better one.

Not being in control of your environment

It is very hard to change an established habit when you aren't in control of what is happening around you. For example, if you are still going out to the local greasy spoon with your colleagues at lunch every day, losing those 15lb before your golfing trip to the Costa del Sol is going to prove very difficult. However, by choosing to have lunch somewhere different that has healthier options, it'll make it easier for you to avoid unhealthy foods.

Don't try to change too many habits at once

When you are looking at HOT and living life optimally, it can be tempting to try and cut out all of your bad habits and trade them for new, healthy ones all at once. However, trying to change too much at once is often a quick route to failure. It's too much pressure and there are too many new things to try and remember. Instead, focus on one at a time.

Check your commitment levels

Changing any habit is a time-consuming process and can require a lot of hard graft. Don't underestimate the commitment you need, and the patience and determination required to achieve the goals you have set for yourself.

Don't focus too much on the result

If you are driven by results, this is something that is going to be tricky, but try not to focus too much on your end goal. Short, interim results like losing half a stone before a holiday are great motivational tools in the beginning, but the goal of Hormone Optimisation Therapy and living life optimally is to inspire long-term positive changes. It's a marathon, not a sprit!

Don't assume major changes are the only changes you can make

Another common mistake is setting the bar too high by opting to make big, loud changes instead of small quiet ones. The trouble is, these are often harder to stick with. For example, rather than saying you will give up smoking completely from tomorrow, try a smaller goal instead such as reducing how much you smoke. It is generally considered much easier to go from 20 cigarettes a day to none at all when you've gradually been reducing the amount you've been having each day over the last six weeks.

My eight step guide to building good habits

1 – Get rid of triggers

Carefully identify the places, people and activities that your mind uses as triggers to initiate bad habits. By changing your behaviour towards those things, you are one step closer to eliminating bad habits from your day to day life. For example, if you crave cakes but are trying to limit your sugar intake, arrange to meet friends for a walk rather than a coffee.

2 - Replace your cravings

Reducing cravings can be easier said than done, but it may be possible to replace them with a healthier or better alternative, such as replacing the relaxing feeling you get from having a glass of wine with having a soak in the bath to create the same feeling of relaxation.

3 – Make it hard to follow your bad habit

When it comes to habits, we are our own worst enemy. Generally, if we think that something is too hard for us to achieve, it puts us off even trying to. But one thing we can do is to make it harder for us to engage with our bad habits.

For example, if our bad habit is nipping out for a smoke with colleagues at 11am, we could schedule a meeting at that time to prevent us from joining them. Or if your bad habit is going to bed too late, you could start setting your alarm clock earlier to make you more tired the next day. Don't be afraid to think outside the box when it comes to coming up with ways to make it hard to follow your bad habits.

4 – Get to the root of the problem

It's not always possible to determine why we develop the habits we do, but if you can get to the bottom of why you do what you do, it could help you to change it. You might find that you drink when you are stressed because you don't have any other coping strategies in place, but by recognising this and looking at alternative ways of coping, such as exercise or meditation, you could swap one bad habit for a better one.

5 – Make your routines healthy

Establishing good habits means making good lifestyle choices. A very good way to accomplish this is by overhauling your routines. As mentioned previously in this section, making small changes can be much more effective than trying to jump straight in the deep end with bigger ones. You'll be surprised just how quickly the little changes can improve your health and happiness.

6 – Swap bad habits for better ones

Yes, I know we've mentioned it before, but it is far easier to swap a bad habit for a good one than cut it out altogether. Look at ways you can make small changes to a habit that you'd like to improve, such as turning notifications off on your phone an hour before bed instead of just before you go to sleep or swapping your usual coffee for a green tea.

7 – Use reminders

In the earliest stages of habit-building, remembering that you are trying to forge and maintain healthy habits is often the most challenging part! Using reminders is one the easiest ways of keeping yourself on track – whether that's post-it notes on your laptop or fridge, or reminders on your phone. There are also plenty of habit-tracking apps available that you can download onto your phone.

8 – Be kind to yourself

We already know that building new habits can be tricky and maintaining them can be even more difficult. If you pressure yourself too much you may find that it is counterproductive. For instance, if you slip up for a few days and miss your morning exercise, you may want to give up altogether. Be kind to yourself and avoid thinking that you are a failure or that you are never going to succeed - that will not help. Simply resolve to do better next week and stick to it.

18.
Gut health and hormones

You've probably heard the phrase "you are what you eat", but you may not realise that when your gut health isn't optimal, your hormonal balance can be thrown out of whack.

A healthy gut will include trillions of microorganisms that live inside a pocket in your large intestine called the cecum, and they all contribute to keep processes like educating the immune system, protecting against pathogens and metabolic function. Low microbial diversity or not having enough different bacteria in your gut has been linked to high thyroid hormone levels and therefore hypothyroidism, a condition often associated with low testosterone levels plus a variety of other illnesses and syndromes [37].

The gut microbiome also influences a kind of bacteria called estrobolome. The primary purpose of estrobolome is to metabolise oestrogen, which as we already know, must be perfectly balanced in both men and women.

Fortunately, there's lots of ways to boost your gut health including:

- Avoiding refined sugar and ditch artificial sweeteners
- Choosing organic food when possible
- Eating lots of vegetables
- Getting good sleep
- Exercising regularly
- Consuming fibre
- Avoiding smoking
- Including probiotics in your diet

This brings me on to the very last part of this little book on Hormone Optimisation Therapy – Paleo.

19.
Paleo

The Paleo diet is designed to resemble what our ancestors ate thousands of years ago, which was basically what they could hunt or gather at the time. Obviously, this varied by geographical region and many of the animals, fruits and vegetables that existed back then have been replaced, but the premise remains focused on a diet of whole, unprocessed foods.

A paleo diet isn't necessarily for everyone. However, studies have found links between following a paleo diet and a lower risk of cardiovascular disease [38]. It's also been suggested that it could be beneficial for weight loss, lowering your blood pressure and cholesterol and boosting energy levels. Finally, it's a diet that I have found to be particularly helpful in keeping me on track when I find that my healthy habits are starting to slip and forms an important part of my HOT plan.

In general, a paleo diet follows these rules:

Foods you can eat
- Fruits
- Vegetables
- Nuts and seeds
- Eggs
- Lean meats, especially grass-fed animals and wild game
- Fish, particularly those rich in omega-3 fatty acids like salmon and mackerel
- Oils from fruits and nuts, like olive oil

Things to avoid
- Grains, like wheat, oat and barley
- Legumes, like beans, lentils and peanuts
- Dairy products, like milk and cheese
- Anything containing refined and added sugar
- Added salt
- Starchy vegetables like peas and white potatoes
- Processed foods like cookies and crisps

There are heaps of resources about paleo diets online, including plenty of recipes, hints and tips. There's also a list of suggested foods included in the appendix of this book.

20.
Epilogue

Whether you are just starting your andropause journey or you've been looking for answers to the way you are feeling for some time, I hope you've found this short book on Hormone Optimisation Therapy helpful. And if you are still keen to learn more about male menopause, testosterone replacement therapy or any of the other elements of this book, please check out our website www.alphagenix.co.uk where you'll find videos, blogs and other resources.

With better understanding, more open conversations and simple, life-optimising lifestyle changes, we can face the future with happiness, confidence and good health.

21.
Signposting

Movember – a leading charity for changing the face of men's mental health.
https://uk.movember.com/about/foundation

Andy's Man Club – a suicide prevention charity, offering free peer-to-peer support groups across the UK and online.
https://andysmanclub.co.uk/

Directions for Men – a male mental health support community.
https://www.directionsformen.org.uk/

22.
Sources

1 https://www.healthline.com/health/low-testosterone/testosterone-levels-by-age#normal-testosterone-levels

2 https://academic.oup.com/jsm/article/14/12/1504/6973374

3 https://www.medichecks.com/blogs/testosterone/why-do-gen-z-and-millennial-men-have-lower-testosterone

4 https://cdn.movember.com/uploads/images/2012/News/UK%20IRE%20ZA/Movember%20Masculinity%20%26%20Opening%20Up%20Report%2008.10.19%20FINAL.pdf

5 https://www.nhs.uk/mental-health/conditions/clinical-depression/symptoms/

6 https://www.addictioncenter.com/addiction/differences-men-women/

7 https://www.healthcentre.org.uk/pharmacy/erectile-dysfunction-statistics.html

8 https://www.ncbi.nlm.nih.gov/pmc/articles/PMC4854098/

9 https://www.ncbi.nlm.nih.gov/pmc/articles/PMC3134227/

10 https://www.webmd.com/men/features/keep-testosterone-in-balance

11 https://www.healthline.com/health/trt

12 https://www.health.harvard.edu/mens-health/is-testosterone-therapy-safe-take-a-breath-before-you-take-the-plunge

13 https://www.health.harvard.edu/mens-health/is-testosterone-therapy-safe-take-a-breath-before-you-take-the-plunge%2012

14 https://paihdelinkki.fi/en/info-bank/articles/medicinal-substances/testosterone-and-anabolic-steroid-abuse-side-effects

15 https://www.kch.nhs.uk/Doc/pl%20-%20934.1%20-%20testosterone%20replacement%20therapy.pdf

16 https://www.ncbi.nlm.nih.gov/pmc/articles/PMC3188848/

17 https://pubmed.ncbi.nlm.nih.gov/33503312/

18 https://www.ncbi.nlm.nih.gov/pmc/articles/PMC3370421/

19 https://edclinics.co.uk/advice/shockwave-therapy-for-ed-at-home/

20 https://medlineplus.gov/genetics/understanding/traits/longevity/

21 https://www.who.int/teams/environment-climate-change-and-health/air-quality-and-health/health-impacts

22 https://www.cornwall.gov.uk/environment/environmental-protection/radon/

23 https://www.hopkinsmedicine.org/health/wellness-and-prevention/special-heart-risks-for-men

24 https://risemenshealth.com/tbi-ptsd-and-low-testosterone/

25 – source for TRT and PTSD from Ross

26 - https://www.health.harvard.edu/staying-healthy/blue-light-has-a-dark-side

27 https://health.ucdavis.edu/blog/cultivating-health/blue-light-effects-on-your-eyes-sleep-and-health/2022/08

28 https://www.ncbi.nlm.nih.gov/pmc/articles/PMC5941775/

29 https://www.webmd.com/skin-problems-and-treatments/red-light-therapy

30 https://www.everydayhealth.com/heart-health/viagra-and-cialis-may-cut-risk-of-early-death-from-heart-disease/

31 https://www.hsph.harvard.edu/nutritionsource/healthy-weight/diet-reviews/intermittent-fasting/

32 https://www.hopkinsmedicine.org/health/wellness-and-prevention/intermittent-fasting-what-is-it-and-how-does-it-work

33 https://www.mayoclinic.org/healthy-lifestyle/stress-management/in-depth/stress/art-20046037

34 https://www.apa.org/topics/mindfulness/meditation

35 https://www.ncbi.nlm.nih.gov/pmc/articles/PMC8992377/

36 https://psychcentral.com/health/need-to-form-a-new-habit

37 https://www.ncbi.nlm.nih.gov/pmc/articles/PMC8990747/

38 https://www.mayoclinic.org/healthy-lifestyle/nutrition-and-healthy-eating/in-depth/paleo-diet/art-20111182

23.
Book Bonus

As a thank you for buying this book, please scan the QR code below, complete your details and recieve a *Free Testosterone Booster Guide*.

For more information contact us here:
https://alphagenix.co.uk/
info@ alphagenix.co.uk

Printed in Great Britain
by Amazon

24987407R00079